Examining New Approaches for Implementing Vaccine Mandates Within the Department of Defense

How Lessons Learned from COVID-19
Vaccine Mandates Could Improve Future
Vaccination Campaigns

DANIEL M. GERSTEIN, TRUPTI BRAHMBHATT,
SAMANTHA CHERNEY, KRISTIE L. GORE

Prepared for the Department of Defense
Approved for public release; distribution unlimited

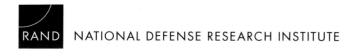

NATIONAL DEFENSE RESEARCH INSTITUTE

For more information on this publication, visit **www.rand.org/t/RRA1829-1**.

About RAND

The RAND Corporation is a research organization that develops solutions to public policy challenges to help make communities throughout the world safer and more secure, healthier and more prosperous. RAND is nonprofit, nonpartisan, and committed to the public interest. To learn more about RAND, visit www.rand.org.

Research Integrity

Our mission to help improve policy and decisionmaking through research and analysis is enabled through our core values of quality and objectivity and our unwavering commitment to the highest level of integrity and ethical behavior. To help ensure our research and analysis are rigorous, objective, and nonpartisan, we subject our research publications to a robust and exacting quality-assurance process; avoid both the appearance and reality of financial and other conflicts of interest through staff training, project screening, and a policy of mandatory disclosure; and pursue transparency in our research engagements through our commitment to the open publication of our research findings and recommendations, disclosure of the source of funding of published research, and policies to ensure intellectual independence. For more information, visit www.rand.org/about/research-integrity.

RAND's publications do not necessarily reflect the opinions of its research clients and sponsors.

Published by the RAND Corporation, Santa Monica, Calif.
© 2023 RAND Corporation
RAND® is a registered trademark.

Library of Congress Cataloging-in-Publication Data is available for this publication.
ISBN: 978-1-9774-1077-1

Cover: James Thew/Adobe Stock.

Limited Print and Electronic Distribution Rights

About This Report

This exploratory report was written in the time of the coronavirus disease 2019 (COVID-19) pandemic in July 2022, some two and a half years after the first cases were identified. Therefore, the impetus for this study was to (1) understand how the Department of Defense (DoD) COVID-19 vaccination program was developed and implemented, (2) determine how previous DoD vaccination programs influenced those decisions, and (3) identify opportunities to strengthen the department's vaccination program, particularly against emerging infectious diseases, such as COVID-19.[1]

The research reported here was completed in July 2022 and underwent security review with the sponsor and the Defense Office of Prepublication and Security Review before public release.

Vaccinations are a complex and emotional subject in the United States. In this report, we do not take a position on specific vaccinations for the U.S. population or DoD military or civilian personnel. Rather, we recognize that vaccinations are an important component of public health. For the military, vaccination policies are a matter of mission readiness and force health protection. It is from this understanding that we wrote this report and made recommendations with respect to future DoD vaccination programs. Finally, we do not address ongoing discussions about the congressional repeal of the COVID-19 vaccination mandate.

RAND National Security Research Division

This research was conducted within the Forces and Resources Policy Program of the RAND National Security Research Division, which operates the RAND National Defense Research Institute (NDRI), a federally funded research and development center (FFRDC) sponsored by the Office of the Secretary of Defense, the Joint Staff, the Unified Combatant Commands, the Navy, the Marine Corps, the defense agencies, and the defense intelligence enterprise. This research was made possible by NDRI exploratory research funding that was provided through the FFRDC contract and approved by NDRI's primary sponsor.

For more information on the RAND Forces and Resources Policy Program, see www.rand.org/nsrd/frp or contact the director (contact information is provided on the webpage).

---

[1] Since the writing of this report, the National Defense Authorization Act for Fiscal Year 2023 (H.R. 7900) was approved on December 8, 2022. Section 525 of this law rescinded the COVID-19 vaccine mandate for members of the U.S. Armed Forces.

Acknowledgments

We would like to acknowledge Laura Baldwin and Molly McIntosh for their foresight in deciding to fund research on this critical topic.

Contents

About This Report iii

Figures and Tables vi

Chapter 1. Introduction 1

    Key Findings 1

    Methodology 1

    The Case for Vaccination 2

Chapter 2. Laws, Regulations, and Policies Governing DoD Vaccinations 6

    Uniform DoD Military Personnel 6

    DoD Civilians and Contractors 8

    Vaccine Status as a Readiness Issue 9

    Overlaps Between Society, Other Government Agencies, and DoD 10

Chapter 3. COVID-19 Vaccine Development and DoD Program, Mandates, and Exemptions ... 12

    COVID-19 Vaccination Requirements 12

    Vaccine Hesitancy 15

    Management of Exemptions for COVID-19 17

    Challenges to Federal Laws 20

Chapter 4. Case Studies: Other DoD Vaccine Campaigns and Mandates 24

    Anthrax Vaccination 24

    Smallpox Vaccination 27

    The Gulf War 29

    "Mandates" as Provision of Work 30

Chapter 5. Observations and Conclusions 32

    Observations and Assessments 32

    Recommendations 35

Abbreviations 37

References 38

Figures and Tables

Figures

Figure 3.1. DoD Vaccine Data (as of May 25, 2022)..17

Figure 5.1. Comparison of Anthrax, Smallpox, and COVID-19 Vaccine Campaigns 34

Tables

Table 2.1. Joint Service Regulation on Immunizations and Chemoprophylaxis for the Prevention of Infectious Diseases..7

Table 3.1. Military Service Vaccination Planning 15

Table 5.1. Proposed Rating Scale for Attributes 33

Chapter 1. Introduction

This report was written in the time of the coronavirus disease 2019 (COVID-19) pandemic in July 2022, some two and a half years after the first cases were identified. Therefore, the impetus for this study was the desire to (1) understand how the Department of Defense (DoD) COVID-19 vaccination program was developed and implemented, (2) determine how previous DoD vaccination programs influenced those decisions, and (3) identify opportunities to strengthen the department's vaccination program, particularly against emerging infectious diseases, such as COVID-19. To that end, we examine the laws and policies that guide the overall DoD vaccination program, study lessons learned from other DoD vaccination programs, and determine the policies for handling medical and administrative (including religious) exemptions. Through this analysis, we can clearly see how the two imperatives of ensuring force health protection and mission readiness have guided and continue to guide the decisions made concerning DoD vaccine policies.

Key Findings

- DoD has a well-founded and well-documented vaccination program that dates to the earliest times of U.S. military history.
- Decisions about DoD vaccine policies regarding COVID-19 were inextricably linked with and dependent on the broader U.S. guidance that came from civilian authorities, such as the Department of Health and Human Services (HHS), Centers for Disease Control and Prevention (CDC), and Food and Drug Administration (FDA).
- The two primary drivers for all DoD decisions were force health protection and mission readiness.
- Comparing three DoD mandatory vaccine programs—for smallpox, anthrax, and COVID-19—demonstrates that perceptions can contribute positively or negatively to the acceptability of mandatory vaccines.
- A RAND Corporation–developed exploratory framework provides six key attributes for consideration in establishing a mandatory vaccine policy: (1) approval status of vaccine, (2) targeting groups for vaccines, (3) consistent messaging, (4) confidence in the technology, (5) disinformation surrounding the vaccine, and (6) perceived care in making decisions about mandates.

Methodology

To examine the interplay between DoD's policies and directives and the civilian authorities that provided the approval for medical countermeasures, including vaccines, we relied on literature searches as the primary source of input. These searches include literature from three primary sources: (1) peer-reviewed literature from such organizations as the Congressional

1

Research Service and Government Accountability Office, as well as from scientific and technical journal articles, (2) news reports on topical issues related to vaccine development, decisionmaking, and mandates and (3) public-facing U.S. government sources, including general historical vaccination information and COVID-19–specific sources, policies, and guidelines.

We looked at the history of vaccine requirements in the military, including initial entry requirements, the special smallpox and anthrax vaccination programs, and vaccines mandated as a provision of work. In doing so, we sought to understand how the status of the vaccine (e.g., Investigational New Drug [IND], which provides approval for clinical trials, Emergency Use Authorization [EUA], and full use), the relationship to the military (e.g., uniformed, DoD civilian, or contractor), and personnel circumstances (e.g., age and medical history) contribute to the necessity (e.g., legal, ethical, or regulatory compliance) of getting vaccinated.

Through analysis of the history of vaccines in the military and several case studies, we draw observations, identify lessons learned, and develop recommendations for improving the military vaccination program. The recommendations are based on our observations and analysis of other military vaccination programs. We have created an exploratory framework as part of these conclusions for considering vaccine acceptability—including the key attributes of a vaccination campaign—which could provide an important basis for thinking about how to manage future DoD vaccination campaigns.

The focus of our report is on the period that begins with the development of the COVID-19 vaccination concept and program to the implementation of the vaccine mandate through the end of June 2022. We have not continued to update the statistics on vaccinations or assessed any policy changes that have occurred since COVID-19 (and its variants) have become globally endemic.

The Case for Vaccination

The U.S. military has a long history of vaccinating service members against infectious disease as a military necessity to protect soldiers and contribute to the overall mission readiness of the force. The military necessity for vaccination became clear with the devastation of the Continental Army in 1776, when over half of the soldiers became ill with smallpox. The following year, General George Washington, the commander-in-chief of the Continental Army, "ordered mandatory inoculation against smallpox for any soldier who had not gained prior immunity against the disease through infection."[1]

Beginning with this first vaccination of soldiers, the U.S. military would rely on an increasingly robust vaccine program to protect the force and preserve its fighting strength. Even in these early days of vaccines, the link between force readiness and vaccines was evident. The

---

[1] College of Physicians of Philadelphia, "U.S. Military and Vaccine History," webpage, undated. It is noteworthy that Washington's directive occurred two decades before Edward Jenner developed his successful cowpox-based vaccine for smallpox.

smallpox vaccination program demonstrates this linkage. One historical account assesses that, had mandatory variolation been performed on the force a year earlier, the smallpox outbreak experienced by the Continental Army could have been avoided, the retreat of the Continental Army from Quebec would not have been necessary, and the end of the Revolutionary War might have been hastened.[2]

As military operations continued to expand and soldiers became exposed to a wide variety of infectious diseases, the military's vaccine program also expanded, in terms of both the number of mandatory vaccines that would be required for the force and the establishment of the military as a leader in vaccine development. The list of vaccines developed by the military grew to include yellow fever as a result of U.S. experiences during the Spanish-American War of 1898, an adenovirus vaccine developed in 1956 following experiences in World War II with respiratory diseases, and an Ebola vaccine following the 2014 outbreak in West Africa, as well as HIV and malaria vaccine research that continues today.[3] Although the U.S. military's vaccine development is beyond the scope of this report, such development demonstrates DoD's continued commitment to disease prevention and protection using vaccines.

Today, the list of mandatory vaccinations required for military personnel upon accession is comprehensive and specifically includes "Service personnel in enlisted initial entry training, Reserve Officers Training Corps (ROTC), Officer Candidate School, academy preparatory school, [and] Service academy."[4]

SARS-CoV-2, the virus that causes COVID-19, has once again demonstrated the importance of the health of the force and readiness. The need to protect the U.S. Armed Forces (and their families) against a virus with such morbidity and mortality rates was imperative to preserve the military's mission readiness. As of May 2022, COVID-19 had killed more than 1 million Americans. Although the number of service members who have died from COVID-19 remains relatively small among this generally fit population,[5] the effects of readiness were felt from the earliest days of the pandemic during the outbreak on the *U.S.S. Theodore Roosevelt* aircraft carrier with 4,779 personnel on board.[6] The *Roosevelt* became mission ineffective and had to be taken off mission and ordered to Guam. The result was that COVID-19 "infected more than

[2] College of Physicians of Philadelphia, undated.

[3] Headquarters, Departments of the Army, the Navy, the Air Force, and the Coast Guard, *Immunizations and Chemoprophylaxis for the Prevention of Infectious Diseases*, October 7, 2013, p. 29.

[4] Headquarters, Departments of the Army, the Navy, the Air Force, and the Coast Guard, 2013, p. 10.

[5] Pete Riley, Michal Ben-Nun, James Turtle, David Bacon, Akeisha N. Owens, and Steven Riley, "COVID-19: On the Disparity in Outcomes Between Military and Civilian Populations," *Military Medicine*, Vol. 188, No. 1–2, January–February 2023.

[6] Ananya Mandal, "COVID-19 Outbreak on an American Aircraft Carrier: A Case Study in Transmission," News Medical, November 16, 2020.

1,200 sailors and killed one, leading to the firing of its captain and the resignation of the Navy's top official."[7]

COVID-19 Vaccine

In January 2020, when the first SARS-CoV-2 isolates became available, a global race to develop a vaccine against the new coronavirus variant began. Two early leaders in this effort were Moderna and Pfizer, with vaccines that use an approach employing messenger RNA technology. By July 14 and August 12, respectively, Moderna and Pfizer published their Phase I and II clinical trial data, which looked promising.[8] Russia and China, as well as several other nations, developed their vaccine candidates using traditional vaccine platforms. By November 2020, several vaccine candidates under development had progressed to clinical trials.[9]

In December 2020, both Moderna and Pfizer received an EUA from the FDA.[10] In describing the rationale for and limits of an EUA, one source states that

> emergency use authorization (EUA) is a tool the Food and Drug Administration (FDA) can use to expedite the availability of medical products, including drugs and vaccines, during a public health emergency. An EUA can only be granted when no adequate, approved, available alternatives exist, and when the known and potential benefits outweigh the potential risks. An EUA also only lasts as long as the public health emergency for which it was declared.[11]

An EUA specifically "requires that vaccine recipients or their caregivers are provided with certain vaccine-specific EUA information to help make an informed decision about vaccination."[12] With the granting of the Moderna and Pfizer EUA, vaccine development (which normally takes ten to 15 years), testing, and approval had been reduced to less than one year.[13] Johnson & Johnson (J&J) received EUA for its COVID-19 vaccine on February 26, 2021.[14]

---

[7] Mary Van Beusekom, "COVID-19 Spread Freely Aboard USS Theodore Roosevelt, Report Shows," Center for Infectious Disease Research and Policy, October 1, 2020.

[8] Will Brothers, "A Timeline of COVID-19 Vaccine Development," BioSpace, December 3, 2020.

[9] It is important to note that the various efforts underway were developed under different levels of transparency in terms of the safety and efficacy of the vaccine candidates. The two U.S. messenger RNA vaccines being developed received great scrutiny but were also very transparent. The same can be said for the Johnson & Johnson vaccine, which used an adenovirus platform. This was not the case for the Chinese- and Russian-developed vaccines, which did not provide details on the results of their clinical trials. Furthermore, the science behind the vaccines and the distribution of vaccines both in the United States and globally are beyond the scope of this report.

[10] Brothers, 2020.

[11] Carrie MacMillan, "Emergency Use Authorization vs. Full FDA Approval: What's the Difference?" Yale Medicine, March 7, 2022.

[12] CDC, "COVID-19 Vaccine Emergency Use Authorization (EUA) Fact Sheets for Recipients and Caregivers," webpage, undated-c.

[13] Brothers, 2020.

[14] J&J, "Johnson & Johnson COVID-19 Vaccine Authorized by U.S. FDA for Emergency Use—First Single-Shot Vaccine in Fight Against Global Pandemic," press release, February 27, 2021.

In September 2021, President Joe Biden issued Executive Order 14043, requiring all federal employees to be vaccinated against COVID-19.[15] On October 18, 2021, the Secretary of Defense issued a COVID-19 vaccine mandate that included all sectors of DoD, including civilians, active duty, Ready Reserve, and National Guard.[16] It is worth emphasizing that because the COVID-19 vaccines at that time were approved under EUA by the FDA, they had not been granted full FDA approval when DoD mandated vaccination.

---

[15] White House, "Executive Order on Requiring Coronavirus Disease 2019 Vaccination for Federal Employees," September 9, 2021.

[16] Gilbert R. Cisneros, Jr., Under Secretary of Defense for Personnel and Readiness, "Force Health Protection Guidance (Supplement 23) Revision 1—Department of Defense Guidance for Coronavirus Disease 2019 Vaccination Attestation, Screening Testing, and Vaccination Verification," memorandum for senior Pentagon leadership, commanders of the combatant commands, and defense agency and DoD field activity directors, October 18, 2021.

Chapter 2. Laws, Regulations, and Policies Governing DoD Vaccinations

There is a long history of requiring service members, DoD civilians, and contractors to maintain up-to-date immunizations upon accession or deployment.

Vaccination guidance is based on DoD Office of Health Affairs assessments, force health protection imperatives, and overall mission and theater threat assessments. The guidance represents both the assessments of the Office of Health Affairs and that of the combatant commander. DoD follows the recommendations of the CDC and the Advisory Committee on Immunization Practices (ACIP) for its vaccination requirements.[17] The ACIP, which includes DoD participants, is a group of "medical and public health experts who develop recommendations on the use of vaccines in the civilian population of the United States."[18]

Requirements fall into three categories: vaccinations during initial entry or basic training; routine adult vaccinations; and special risk-based, or occupation-specific, vaccinations.[19] Although some requirements depend on whether the individual is DoD uniformed personnel, a civilian employee, or a contractor, many of the requirements depend on whether the individual is deployed overseas, regardless of their employment status. These requirements are established in DoD Instruction 6205.02 and laid out in a Joint Service Regulation.[20]

Uniform DoD Military Personnel

Nine immunizations are required for all military personnel, active duty and reserve, as part of the adult routine schedule or upon accession, including "Service personnel in enlisted initial entry training, Reserve Officers Training Corps (ROTC), Officer Candidate School, academy preparatory school, [and] Service academy."[21] Credit is given for all immunizations already received.[22]

Eight of the nine vaccinations are required either upon accession or as part of the adult routine immunization schedule. They are hepatitis A; hepatitis B; influenza; measles, mumps,

---

[17] DoD Instruction 6205.02, *DoD Immunization Program*, U.S. Department of Defense, July 23, 2019, p. 3.

[18] CDC, "Advisory Committee on Immunization Practices (ACIP): General Committee-Related Information," webpage, undated-a.

[19] Bryce H. P. Mendez, "Defense Health Primer: Military Vaccinations," Congressional Research Service, IF11816, updated August 6, 2021a.

[20] Headquarters, Departments of the Army, the Navy, the Air Force, and the Coast Guard, 2013.

[21] Headquarters, Departments of the Army, the Navy, the Air Force, and the Coast Guard, 2013, pp. 10–11.

[22] Headquarters, Departments of the Army, the Navy, the Air Force, and the Coast Guard, 2013, p. 9.

and rubella (MMR); meningococcal; poliovirus; tetanus-diphtheria; and varicella. These are required for the Army, Navy, Air Force, Marine Corps, and Coast Guard.[23] The vaccination for adenovirus is not typically recommended for routine administration in the general population but is given upon initial entry or basic training to DoD service members.[24] These routine or accession vaccinations are distinct to service members; there is no requirement for civilians or contractors to be vaccinated upon hiring. Table 2.1 summarizes the requirements of the DoD vaccination program.

Table 2.1. Joint Service Regulation on Immunizations and Chemoprophylaxis for the Prevention of Infectious Diseases

Table D–1
Immunizations for military personnel

Name of vaccine	Army	Navy	Air Force	Marine Corps	Coast Guard
Adenovirus[1]	Acc[2]	Acc	Acc	Acc	Acc
Anthrax	Risk	Risk	Risk	Risk	Risk
Haemophilus influenzae type b	Risk	Risk	Risk	Risk	Risk
Hepatitis A	Acc, Rou[3]	Acc, Rou	Acc, Rou	Acc, Rou	Acc, Rou
Hepatitis B	Acc, Rou	Acc, Rou	Acc, Rou	Acc, Rou	Acc, Rou
Influenza	Acc, Rou	Acc, Rou	Acc, Rou	Acc, Rou	Acc, Rou
Japanese encephalitis	Risk[4]	Risk	Risk	Risk	Risk
Measles, mumps, rubella	Acc, Rou	Acc, Rou	Acc, Rou	Acc, Rou	Acc, Rou
Meningococcal	Acc, Rou	Acc, Rou	Acc, Rou	Acc, Rou	Acc, Rou
Pneumococcal	Risk	Risk	Risk	Risk	Risk
Poliovirus[5]	Acc, Rou	Acc, Rou	Acc, Rou	Acc, Rou	Acc, Rou
Rabies	Risk	Risk	Risk	Risk	Risk
Smallpox (vaccinia)	Risk	Risk	Risk	Risk	Risk
Tetanus-diphtheria (preferably with pertussis vaccine)	Acc, Rou	Acc, Rou	Acc, Rou	Acc, Rou	Acc, Rou
Typhoid fever	Risk	Risk	Risk	Risk	Risk
Varicella	Acc, Rou	Acc, Rou	Acc, Rou	Acc, Rou	Acc, Rou
Yellow fever	Risk	Risk	Risk	Acc, Risk	Risk

Notes:
[1] Initial entry and basic training accessions only
[2] Acc=accessions
[3] Rou=adult routine
[4] Risk=special, risk-based, and occupational
[5] Refer to paragraph 4–13.

SOURCE: Reproduced from Headquarters, Departments of the Army, the Navy, the Air Force, and the Coast Guard, 2013, p. 29.

---

[23] Headquarters, Departments of the Army, the Navy, the Air Force, and the Coast Guard, 2013, p. 29.

[24] Headquarters, Departments of the Army, the Navy, the Air Force, and the Coast Guard, 2013, p. 29.

Other vaccinations are administered to DoD service members depending on the specific occupational risk or geographic area of deployment. For example, DoD Instruction 6205.02 explains that smallpox and anthrax vaccinations "are restricted to DoD personnel or groups identified by the Office of the Secretary of Defense, in consultation with the [Chairman of the Joint Chiefs of Staff], the Under Secretary of Defense for Intelligence, and the geographic [combatant commanders]."

According to DoD clarifying guidance, anthrax vaccination is required for all personnel assigned to or deploying to the U.S. Central Command (CENTCOM) theater for 15 or more days, and both smallpox and anthrax vaccinations are required for all personnel assigned to or deploying to the Korean Peninsula for 15 or more days. Additionally, both vaccinations are required for "personnel performing duties or services that support the Chemical, Biological, Radiological, and Nuclear Response Enterprises."[25]

Specific requirements are maintained in policies promulgated by individual geographic combatant commands that are updated as necessary. For example, in April 2020, CENTCOM updated the routine and accession vaccinations required, adding that (1) an anthrax vaccination was required for all personnel traveling in the CENTCOM theater for 15 or more days, (2) smallpox vaccination was no longer required, and (3) pre-exposure vaccination was required for individuals working in specific high-risk occupations, including veterinary personnel, dog handlers, and certain laboratory personnel.[26]

DoD Civilians and Contractors

As with service members, civilian DoD employees and DoD contractors receive either country-specific or occupation-specific immunizations.[27] As referenced above, each geographic combatant command promulgates policies for all personnel who travel to theater, and these requirements are the same for service members, civilians, and contractors.[28] The Defense Health Agency outlines all immunization requirements by area of responsibility,[29] which are referenced in geographic combatant command policy memoranda.[30]

---

[25] Deputy Secretary of Defense, "Clarifying Guidance for Smallpox and Anthrax Vaccine Immunization Program," memorandum, November 12, 2015, p. 2.

[26] CENTCOM, "USCENTCOM 091923Z Apr 20 Mod Fifteen to USCENTCOM Individual Protection and Individual-Unit Deployment Policy," 2020, p. 12. Additional information on DoD general health issues, including vaccination policies, can be found at Military Health System, homepage, undated.

[27] DoD Instruction 6205.02, 2019, pp. 12–13; Headquarters, Departments of the Army, the Navy, the Air Force, and the Coast Guard, 2013, pp. 11–12.

[28] See, e.g., CENTCOM, 2020, p. 12.

[29] Defense Health Agency, "Vaccine Recommendations by AOR," webpage, undated.

[30] CENTCOM, 2020, p. 11.

Vaccine Status as a Readiness Issue

Vaccine status is indeed a readiness issue. Disease in warfare typically killed more service members than combat did prior to the understanding of disease and modern medical countermeasures (in particular, vaccines for prevention and treatment using antibiotics).[31] In World War I, 116,516 U.S. service members died, of which some 63,000 service members died from disease, which equates to almost 55 percent of the casualties.[32] With improvements in general health, the use of vaccines, and the advent of sulfonamides and then antibiotics, deaths caused by infection in World War II were reduced to 10 percent (or one in ten) for U.S. service members.[33]

To ensure force health protection and mission readiness, commanders conduct periodic readiness processing for their units. As an example, the Army requires unit commanders to conduct soldier readiness processing (SRP) to ensure that service members, DoD civilians, and contractors who support the military are prepared to deploy.[34] Depending on the unit of assignment, SRPs may be conducted only for predeployment or for units on high alert, which may have to deploy more rapidly, either quarterly or semiannually. A full SRP includes updating security clearances, personnel actions to account for fact-of-life changes (e.g., marriages, births, divorces), and medical, legal, financial, and dental records. As part of the medical stations of the SRP, shot records are examined to ensure that deployable personnel have the necessary vaccinations for the theater to which they are deploying.[35] Vaccination policy and guidance is based on DoD Office of the Assistant Secretary of Defense for Health Affairs and Defense Health Agency assessments, force health protection imperatives, and overall theater threat assessments. The guidance represents the assessments of the Office of Health Affairs and that of the combatant commander. Each of the services has similar SRP requirements for its units.

Efficiently processing large units requires having stations set up for each of the key areas where key post, camp, or station support personnel can be available to provide the needed services. For the medical portion of an SRP, the local hospital or clinic normally provides an immunization station at the processing site. This can include updating the nine immunizations that are required for all military personnel, as well as the theater-specific requirements.

---

[31] Vincent J. Cirillo, "Two Faces of Death: Fatalities from Disease and Combat in America's Principal Wars, 1775 to Present," *Perspectives in Biology and Medicine*, Vol. 51, No. 1, Winter 2008.

[32] Carol R. Byerly, "War Losses (USA)," in Ute Daniel, Peter Gatrell, Oliver Janz, Heather Jones, Jennifer Keene, Alan Kramer, and Bill Nasson, eds., *1914–1918 Online: International Encyclopedia of the First World War*, Freie Universität Berlin, 2014.

[33] Peter C. Doherty, "Stealth Attack: Infection and Disease on the Battlefield," *The Conversation*, June 8, 2015.

[34] I Corps Regulation 600-8-101, *Soldier Readiness Program (SRP)*, Headquarters, I Corps, undated.

[35] This SRP checklist comes from Fort Stewart-Hunter Army Airfield and is representative of what a post would provide for the units that are stationed there. Often, these SRP checklists can be tailored if there are specific requirements established by local commanders or the combatant commander where the unit is to be deployed (Fort Stewart-Hunter Army Airfield, "Soldier Readiness Processing," webpage, undated).

A service member is nondeployable until certain requirements, including vaccinations, have been completed. Therefore, if a soldier is missing a vaccination, they will not be able to deploy. DoD civilians or contractors joining the unit can be included in the SRP to ensure they are prepared to deploy.

Overlaps Between Society, Other Government Agencies, and DoD

Although we directly consider DoD vaccine issues (in particular, for COVID-19) in this report, we must also recognize the interplay between DoD and other entities. Indeed, many overlaps exist between vaccine requirements for use in civil society and within DoD.

For example, DoD laboratories are governed by international agreements, such as the World Health Organization's International Health Regulations (IHR) and the Biological and Toxin Weapons Convention (BWC), as well as member-state national laws. These national laws originate from the IHR and BWC requirements and suggest policies and regulations concerning the handling of biological pathogens.

As a result, DoD laboratories would be governed by the same select agent laws, policies, and regulations as other organizations or individuals. This means that DoD facilities will have regular inspections of high-containment laboratories that deal with human, plant, or animal pathogens. Furthermore, competent authorities from either HHS for human pathogens or the U.S. Department of Agriculture (USDA) for zoonotic pathogens would inspect DoD facilities, including the biosafety and biosecurity of DoD laboratories. Part of these biosafety and biosecurity inspections includes the safety of the researchers and workers at these laboratory facilities, including their vaccination status for those who work with biological pathogens. It would be very unlikely to see vaccine guidance that diverges greatly between DoD, the CDC in HHS, or the Animal and Plant Health Inspection Service in the USDA.

Another important consideration in any vaccination program concerns the *status* of the vaccines: in other words, relating to where a vaccine (or vaccine candidate) is within its life cycle toward meeting its legal, policy, and regulatory requirements for licensure. In this developmental process, vaccines that are regulated by the FDA "undergo a rigorous review of laboratory and clinical data to ensure the safety, efficacy, purity and potency of these products."[36] An important part of this process throughout the vaccine's life cycle is to identify and address any questions of the "vaccine's safety, effectiveness or possible side effects" that arise.[37] There are important differences between vaccines that are fully approved for use versus those for which an IND application has been submitted; pre-licensure vaccine clinical trials for Phases I, II, and III; or even for an EUA vaccine (such as for COVID-19). Even fully approved vaccines can come with warnings for certain groups of people to take precautions or even abstain

---

[36] FDA, "Vaccines," webpage, undated.

[37] FDA, undated.

from taking them. These warnings usually are based on such factors as age or medical history (e.g., allergies, immunocompromised people, or pregnancy). Generally speaking, DoD follows the guidance of the responsible civilian authorities in developing its vaccination guidance and programs.

Chapter 3. COVID-19 Vaccine Development and DoD Program, Mandates, and Exemptions

DoD closely followed the guidance and policies of the competent civilian authorities with responsibility for COVID-19 vaccine development. DoD was certainly a participant in the process, with several direct and indirect touch points along the way. For example, as highlighted previously, DoD participates on the ACIP, which directly influenced COVID-19 vaccine decisions. The initial DoD vaccine guidance adhered closely to the CDC guidance on prioritization of various demographic groups, although DoD had the authority to make exceptions based on mission requirements.

For the armed services and those who support the force, vaccine status became a matter of mission readiness and force health protection. As vaccines became more widely available, these vaccine requirements extended to federal employees. Overall, a small percentage of the military and federal workforce objected to getting the vaccine. As a result, both the military vaccine program mandate and the federal employee executive order would be challenged in the courts.

COVID-19 Vaccination Requirements

A Congressional Research Service report concluded that throughout the military's development of its COVID-19 vaccine policy, "DoD has implemented a variety of conditions-based FHP [force health protection] measures that mirror the U.S. Centers for Disease Control and Prevention's recommended protective measures, to limit the spread of COVID-19 among military personnel."[38] In fact, the DoD vaccine policy has at all times been consistent with and informed by the senior civilian health and regulatory authorities responsible for vaccine policies in the United States.

U.S. efforts to develop COVID-19 vaccines began with the first SARS-CoV-2 isolates that were made available in early January 2020. To coordinate these efforts, the federal government established Operation Warp Speed (OWS) officially on May 15, 2020. OWS represented a partnership on several levels: a partnership between HHS and DoD, a public-private partnership between the federal government and industry, and a partnership between the federal government and state and local governments.[39] OWS initially selected six candidate vaccines that employed several strategies for promoting immunological response. Two of the candidates—Moderna's

---

[38] Bryce H. P. Mendez, "The Military's COVID-19 Vaccination Mandate," Congressional Research Service, IN11764, updated November 8, 2021b, p. 1.

[39] U.S. Government Accountability Office, *Operation Warp Speed: Accelerated COVID-19 Vaccine Development Status and Efforts to Address Manufacturing Challenges*, GAO-21-319, February 11, 2021.

and Pfizer/BioNTech's messenger RNA vaccines—had received FDA approval for EUA in December 2020.[40] Five of the six OWS vaccine candidates had entered Phase III clinical trials as of January 30, 2021.

A J&J vaccine received EUA on February 27, 2021,[41] although the provisions of the EUA were updated one year later as a result of concerns about adverse reactions, including unusual blood clotting, which limited the use of this vaccine product.[42] The messenger RNA vaccines also had some "contraindications and precautions," although these did little to change the applicability or dosing instructions for the Moderna and Pfizer/BioNTech vaccines.[43]

In September 2020, the National Academies of Sciences, Engineering, and Medicine released draft guidelines "to assist policymakers in planning for an equitable allocation of a vaccine against COVID-19." Foundational principles for the allocation of early vaccines included the risks of acquiring infection, severe morbidity and mortality, negative societal impact, and transmitting disease to others.[44] The final National Academies report recommended a four-phase protocol, beginning with the most vulnerable and most crucial workers in society and, in the final stage, including the entire U.S. population (minus those with underlying conditions and those with approved exemptions).[45] Military members and veterans were prioritized within these allocation guidelines in terms of their duties (e.g., as health care workers), their health status (i.e., comorbidities), or if a deployment was imminent.

During the early stages of the COVID-19 vaccination program, the vaccines were voluntary, although some employers required their employees to be vaccinated as a provision of their work status. For example, some hospitals required COVID-19 vaccines for health care workers.[46] However, by and large, vaccines were considered voluntary; for those who were vaccinated, the use of masks became optional. The mask guidance based on vaccine status was ambiguous, sometimes inconsistent, challenging to implement and enforce, and implemented unevenly across the country. There were differences in guidance for those who worked in a federal building, in state government, and in the private sector, all living in the same state. This continued through the end of August 2021 because of fact-of-life changes that altered DoD vaccine policy: the emergence of the Delta variant and the change in vaccine status.

---

[40] U.S. Government Accountability Office, 2021.

[41] J&J, 2021.

[42] CDC, "Janssen (Johnson & Johnson) COVID-19 Vaccine," webpage, undated-f.

[43] CDC, undated-f.

[44] National Academies of Sciences, Engineering, and Medicine, "National Academies Release Draft Framework for Equitable Allocation of a COVID-19 Vaccine, Seek Public Comment," press release, September 1, 2020a.

[45] National Academies of Sciences, Engineering, and Medicine, "National Academies Release Framework for Equitable Allocation of a COVID-19 Vaccine for Adoption by HHS, State, Tribal, Local, and Territorial Authorities," press release, October 2, 2020b.

[46] Carla Delgado, "More Hospitals Are Now Mandating COVID-19 Vaccines for Healthcare Workers," Verywell Health, July 30, 2021.

The Delta variant became the dominant variant of the virus in August 2021. This variant was highly contagious and led to a rapid rise in cases and hospitalizations.[47] The Secretary of Defense's August 24, 2021, memorandum—which came after the FDA approved the Pfizer-BioNTech COVID-19 vaccine a day earlier for individuals 16 years or older—directed the secretaries of the military departments to "immediately begin full vaccination of all members of the Armed Forces under DoD authority on active duty or in the Ready Reserve, including the National Guard, who are not fully vaccinated against COVID-19."[48] In accordance with DoD's overall vaccine exemption policies, service members could request either administrative or medical exemptions from mandatory vaccinations.

Almost two weeks later, on September 9, 2021, President Biden signed the "Executive Order on Requiring Coronavirus Disease 2019 Vaccination for Federal Employees," stating that "to promote the health and safety of the federal workforce and the efficiency of the civil service, it is necessary to require COVID-19 vaccination for all Federal employees subject to such exceptions as required by law."[49] The executive order emphasized the vaccine status of the three "available" vaccines, stating that

> the Pfizer-BioNTech COVID-19 Vaccine, also known as Comirnaty, has received approval from the Food and Drug Administration (FDA), and two others, the Moderna COVID-19 Vaccine and the Janssen COVID-19 Vaccine, have been authorized by the FDA for emergency use. The FDA has determined that all three vaccines meet its rigorous standards for safety, effectiveness, and manufacturing quality.[50]

Citing President Biden's executive order, DoD expanded on its August 24, 2021 service member vaccine directive by adding DoD civilian employees to the department's vaccine mandate program in an October 4, 2021, press release. It required that "all DoD civilian employees must be fully vaccinated by November 22, 2021, subject to exemptions as required by law."[51]

Throughout the vaccine development and deployment, guidance continued to evolve as new information or approvals became available. Clinical trials further determined the safety and efficacy of modified vaccines for new age groups, resulting in additional FDA approvals. Through monitoring of the vaccination program, the FDA identified issues that resulted in new

---

[47] Paul A. Christensen, Randall J. Olsen, S. Wesley Long, Sishir Subedi, James J. Davis, Parsa Hodjat, Debbie R. Walley, Jacob C. Kinskey, Matthew Ojeda Saavedra, Layne Pruitt, et al., "Delta Variants of SARS-CoV-2 Cause Significantly Increased Vaccine Breakthrough COVID-19 Cases in Houston, Texas," *American Journal of Pathology*, Vol. 192, No. 2, February 2022.

[48] Mendez, 2021b.

[49] White House, 2021.

[50] White House, 2021.

[51] DoD, "Mandatory Coronavirus Disease 2019 Vaccination of DoD Civilian Employees," press release, October 4, 2021.

guidance. For example, the FDA called for a pause in the use of the J&J vaccines in April 2021 to investigate instances of blood clotting and added a warning label for the vaccine in July 2021 based on reported cases of Guillain-Barré syndrome in vaccine recipients.[52] The FDA also expanded its guidance on its definition of *fully vaccinated* for each of the approved vaccines.

It is important to consider that the DoD COVID-19 vaccination program did not exist in isolation. As a result, the DoD guidance to the force, both military service members and federal civilians, reflected the guidance of the HHS, CDC, and FDA. Furthermore, the concerns of the DoD populations mirrored those of the general population at large, albeit with far less frequency, likely because of DoD's mandatory, more stringent vaccine requirements for a broad range of infectious diseases as part of initial entry into the military.

The Secretary of Defense's August 24, 2021, memorandum charged each of the services with developing an implementation plan. Table 3.1 provides the vaccination plan by component (i.e., active, reserve, National Guard) for each of the services.

Table 3.1. Military Service Vaccination Planning

Military Service	Component	Date
Army	Active Component	December 15, 2021
	Reserve Component	June 30, 2022
	National Guard	June 30, 2022
Air Force	Active Component	November 2, 2021
	Reserve Component	December 2, 2021
	National Guard	December 2, 2021
Coast Guard	Active Component	Immediately, as soon as operations allow
	Reserve Component	Immediately, as soon as operations allow
Marine Corps	Active Component	November 28, 2021
	Reserve Component	December 28, 2021
Navy	Active Component	November 28, 2021
	Reserve Component	December 28, 2021
Space Force	Active Component	November 2, 2021

SOURCE: Features information from Mendez, 2021b, p. 3.

Vaccine Hesitancy

The national debate about the safety and efficacy of vaccines that were perceived to be rushed to meet the demands of the COVID-19 pandemic resulted in vaccine hesitancy that remains as of this writing. Vaccine hesitancy was amplified by disinformation regarding how the

---

[52] Erika Edwards, "FDA Adds Warning to J&J Vaccine for Possible Link to Rare Neurological Disorder," *NBC News*, July 12, 2021.

vaccine was developed (e.g., use of fetal tissue), use of unproven technology (e.g., use of messenger RNA vaccines), concerns about clinical trials (e.g., based on the wide range of opinions expressed during public debates about safety and efficacy by such stakeholders as scientists, the CDC, and the FDA), and conspiracy theories (e.g., using the vaccines for implanting tracking devices). Some populations also expressed concerns because of previous unethical treatment, such as African Americans and the Tuskegee Syphilis Study.[53] Political affiliation also resulted in differences in willingness to get vaccinated, with one September 2021 study indicating that only 4 percent of Democrats would definitely not be planning to get a vaccination, whereas that number was 23 percent for Republicans.[54]

Despite these issues, DoD remains well above national averages for vaccinations. As of October 2021, 95 percent of the 1.4 million active-duty service members had received at least one dose of the COVID-19 vaccine.[55] In comparison, consider that, as of May 2022, only 78 percent of the U.S. population had received one dose, 66 percent were considered fully vaccinated, and 31 percent had received a booster dose.[56]

DoD continues to update its guidance on COVID-2019 force health protection, with its most recent publication in April 2022.[57] Furthermore, DoD continues to track vaccination status for all service members and DoD federal civilians. Figure 3.1 provides the data as of May 25, 2022.[58]

It is noteworthy that as the June 30, 2022, deadline for vaccination in the services approached, the Army reported having 60,000 unvaccinated soldiers, with a majority of those soldiers coming from the Army Reserve and National Guard. A June 24, 2022, *Washington Post* article attributes the shortfalls in vaccination to the "persistent struggle for commanders to bring soldiers under compliance." This amounts to "nearly 12% of Army National Guard and 10% of Army Reserve soldiers." The article states that about 3,400 service members from all services have been removed from the military for COVID-19 vaccine refusal.[59]

---

[53] Elizabeth Nix, "Tuskegee Experiment: The Infamous Syphilis Study," History, December 15, 2020.

[54] Liz Hamel, Lunna Lopes, Grace Sparks, Ashley Kirzinger, Audrey Kearney, Mellisha Stokes, and Mollyann Brodie, "KFF COVID-19 Vaccine Monitor: September 2021," Kaiser Family Foundation, September 28, 2021.

[55] Janet A. Aker, "More Than 95% of Active Duty Have Received COVID-19 Vaccine," Defense Health Agency, October 15, 2021.

[56] USAFacts, "US Coronavirus Vaccine Tracker: What's the Nation's Progress on Vaccinations?" webpage, undated.

[57] DoD, "Consolidated Department of Defense Coronavirus Disease 2019 Force Health Protection Guidance," press release, April 6, 2022.

[58] DoD, "Coronavirus: DOD Response," webpage, undated.

[59] Alex Horton, "As Army Deadline Nears, About 60,000 Part-Time Soldiers Unvaccinated," *Washington Post*, June 24, 2022.

Figure 3.1. DoD Vaccine Data (as of May 25, 2022)

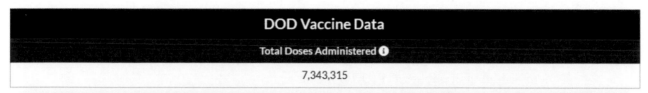

DOD Vaccine Data					
Total Doses Administered ❶					
7,343,315					

DOD Vaccination Data					
	Army	**Marine Corps**	**Navy**	**Air Force ❶**	**Service Member Total**	**DOD Civilian**
Partially Vaccinated	285,211	6,245	6,851	29,756	328,063	50,710
Fully Vaccinated	622,364	195,797	384,944	477,192	1,680,297	341,836

Service member data updated 0600, May 25, 2022*
DOD civilian data updated 0600, November 24, 2021*

*DOD civilian data is as of 0600 November 24, and includes only federal employees who received vaccinations through DOD providers or who are also military health care beneficiaries. The Office of Management and Budget has vaccination data for all DOD federal employees.

Data includes Active Duty, Reserve, and National Guard.

Data is updated weekly. There can be a delay between the time a vaccination record occurs and appears in a health record system.

Partially vaccinated represents the total number of people who received at least one dose of a two-dose COVID-19 vaccine series. Fully vaccinated represents the number of people who have received the second dose in a two-dose COVID-19 vaccine series or one dose of the single-shot Johnson and Johnson Janssen COVID-19 vaccine.

SOURCE: Reproduced from DoD, undated.

Management of Exemptions for COVID-19

The COVID-19 vaccination program follows the same protocols and guidance as other DoD mandatory vaccines, including the use of EUA vaccines and requests for exemptions. The guidance is promulgated in the *Immunizations and Chemoprophylaxis for the Prevention of Infectious Diseases*, which is a DoD publication. The guidance specifies two types of exemptions: immunization-medical and administrative. The broad guidance governing these two exemption categories states, "Granting medical exemptions is a medical function. Granting administrative exemptions is a nonmedical function."[60]

The 2022 National Defense Authorization Act also contains specific language regarding COVID-19 vaccinations. Section 717 requires DoD to track and record information on vaccine

---

[60] Headquarters, Departments of the Army, the Navy, the Air Force, and the Coast Guard, 2013, p. 6.

17

administration. Section 720 is the more pertinent of the sections regarding the exemption issue and requires establishing

> uniform procedures under which covered members may be exempted from receiving an otherwise mandated COVID-19 vaccine for administrative, medical, or religious reasons, including on the basis of possessing an antibody test result demonstrating previous COVID-19 infection.[61]

Medical Exemptions

Health care providers are charged with deciding whether there is a "medical contraindication" regarding the administering of a specific vaccine to a service member. Competent medical authorities can grant "temporary (up to 365 days) or permanent" exemption status. Such a determination can be based on identifying underlying health conditions, evidence of prior immunity, or where the "clinical case is not definable."[62] The regulation allows for obtaining a second opinion if necessary and can be revoked when the exemption is "no longer clinically warranted."[63]

Medical exemptions are coded according to seven categories. Five of the categories are classified as *indefinite*: (1) declined (for optional vaccines), (2) assumed (for previous immunization inferred), (3) immune (based on evidence of immunity from serologic antibody test), (4) permanent (based on a contraindication such as HIV infection or immune suppression), or (5) reactive (based on a permanent restriction because of a previous severe reaction). The two other exemptions are temporary. The first temporary exemption is for up to 90 days due to a "lack of vaccine supply," and the second is for a temporary condition, such as pregnancy, hospitalization, or temporary immune suppression.[64] Once the rationale for the temporary exemption has been resolved, the service member is expected to receive the necessary vaccination.

The approval authority for medical exemptions varied slightly by service but remained in DoD medical channels. Temporary medical exemptions (less than 365 days) could be granted by the DoD medical provider, whereas permanent medical exemptions (longer that 365 days) were elevated to the regional health command, command surgeon, or flag officer levels.[65]

---

[61] Public Law 117-81, National Defense Authorization Act for Fiscal Year 2022, December 27, 2021.

[62] Headquarters, Departments of the Army, the Navy, the Air Force, and the Coast Guard, 2013, p. 6.

[63] Headquarters, Departments of the Army, the Navy, the Air Force, and the Coast Guard, 2013, p. 6.

[64] Headquarters, Departments of the Army, the Navy, the Air Force, and the Coast Guard, 2013, p. 28.

[65] Mendez, 2021b, p. 3.

Administrative Exemptions

There are eight categories of administrative exemptions, which can be grouped into three general issues.[66] The first issue is related to the unavailability of the individual and includes (1) deceased (indefinite), (2) emergency leave (up to 30 days), (3) missing in action or as a prisoner of war (indefinite), and (4) if the individual has had a permanent change of station and departed the unit (up to 90 days). The second issue involves a change in an individual's eligibility or occupational category that removes the vaccination requirement.

The third issue involves a pending administrative legal action: (1) separation, (2) temporary, or (3) refusal. Service members pending separation could request an exemption, including those service members with a pending administrative discharge within 60 days or within 180 days of retiring. Temporary exemption status would include service members who are absent without leave (AWOL) or pending other legal action other than refusal.

The vaccine refusal category consists of those personnel who have refused the vaccine and are pending actions either under the Uniform Code of Military Justice (UCMJ) or for religious reasons and are pending adjudication of their exemption request. Service members remain in this category until their exemption status is resolved.

It is noteworthy that the exemption categories are not mutually exclusive. In other words, service members can be in multiple categories simultaneously or sequentially. For example, a pregnant soldier could be exempt due to pregnancy and, after giving birth, could refuse the vaccine, thus moving to the administrative refusal category. Likewise, an airman could refuse the vaccine, be pending UCMJ, and go AWOL, placing them in multiple categories simultaneously.

The approval authority for general administrative exemptions (i.e., other than for religious accommodations) was delegated to the unit commander in all services except for the Coast Guard, where it was held at the Chief of Military Personnel Policy at Coast Guard Headquarters. The approval authority for religious accommodations was at either service headquarters (Army, Coast Guard, Marine Corps, Navy) or the major command or field command level (Air Force, Space Force).[67]

Although it is not specifically addressed within the medical or administrative exemption categories, EUA can also be a factor. Medical countermeasures for "chemical, biological, radiological, and nuclear (CBRN) agents or threats" receiving EUA are specifically addressed in the regulation, although the language does not elaborate on whether it pertains to threats or agents that are naturally occurring and/or manmade. A vaccine approved by the FDA for EUA can be granted this status for up to 12 months and can be renewed, as necessary. Furthermore, in

---

[66] The information in this section comes from Headquarters, Departments of the Army, the Navy, the Air Force, and the Coast Guard, 2013, p. 28, unless stated otherwise.

[67] Mendez, 2021b, p. 3.

granting EUA, the FDA "may decide that potential recipients of a drug under an EUA should have the option to refuse it. The President may waive this option for military personnel."[68]

The refusal category is certainly the most complicated exemption to adjudicate. Unlike the medical exemption and other administrative categories, which depend on a documented medical diagnosis or an upcoming change in status and can be objectively assessed, the refusal category on religious grounds requires a more subjective assessment of whether the service member has sincerely held beliefs that would prohibit vaccination.

Challenges to Federal Laws

Despite the overall high vaccination rates among DoD personnel, there have been several legal challenges to the vaccine mandates. In describing the DoD COVID-19 vaccination status, a January 31, 2022, Associated Press account provides the following:

> Thousands of members of the active-duty military and the reserves are seeking medical, administrative or religious exemptions or refusing the shots. But overall, the percentage of troops, particularly active duty members, who quickly got the vaccine is high—with at least 97% in each service getting at least one shot as of last week [beginning January 23, 2022].[69]

The same account highlighted that "nearly 600 Marines, airmen and sailors have been thrown out of the military or dismissed from entry-level training at boot camps as of last week [beginning January 23, 2022]."[70]

However, given that both the Pfizer and Moderna vaccines are fully FDA-approved, and that the J&J vaccine has been FDA-approved for those who cannot receive either of the messenger RNA vaccines or those "willing to get the J&J vaccines,"[71] successfully challenging the DoD vaccine mandate has become far less likely.

DoD Service Member Legal Challenges to the COVID-19 Vaccine Mandate

In October 2021, 23 plaintiffs, comprised of Navy, Air Force, Marine Corps, Army, and National Guard service members, as well as contractors and civilian employees for DoD and the Department of Energy, filed a class action suit against President Biden, Secretary of Defense Lloyd Austin, and Secretary of Homeland Security Alejandro Mayorkas in a Florida district

---

[68] Headquarters, Departments of the Army, the Navy, the Air Force, and the Coast Guard, 2013, p. 21.

[69] Lolita C. Baldor, "Austin to Governors: Guard Troops Must Get COVID-19 Vaccine," Associated Press, January 31, 2022.

[70] Baldor, 2022.

[71] Alyssa Billingsley, "FDA COVID-19 Vaccine Approval: Live Updates on Pfizer, Moderna, and J&J Vaccines," GoodRx Health, updated May 20, 2022.

court.[72] As vaccination deadlines neared, the plaintiffs sought a temporary restraining order, preliminary and permanent injunctions, and declaratory relief to "prevent these military heroes, federal employees, and federal contractors from facing punishments including dishonorable discharge, court martial, other life-altering disciplinary procedures, and termination" and argued that they should not have to choose between dishonorable discharge and "sinning against God."[73] They maintained that the mandate violates the federal Religious Freedom Restoration Act of 1993.[74]

In February 2022, the three groups of plaintiffs were separated into three lawsuits, and two service member plaintiffs were granted preliminary injunctions. In March, the 11th Circuit Court of Appeals upheld the preliminary injunctions and granted a limited partial stay pending appeal. In April, the lower court judged issued a preliminary injunction for a Marine Corps captain and a temporary restraining order for an Air Force cadet.[75]

In a similar case, 35 Navy personnel, including 26 SEALs, filed suit on religious grounds in Texas. In January 2022, a Texas district court issued a preliminary injunction, preventing the Navy from either dismissing or reassigning plaintiffs because of vaccine status. The lawsuit made its way to the Supreme Court, which issued a partial stay in March, preventing the Navy from separating the plaintiffs but ruling that they could be reassigned to nondeployable positions.[76]

Another case that made its way to the Supreme Court is a lawsuit by an Air Force reservist similarly seeking a religious exemption. His request for temporary relief was rejected at the district and appeal courts, and his appeal to the Supreme Court "seeking only to block the Air Force from 'inflicting punishments that deprive him of his First Amendment freedoms and irreparably harm his career, including by categorically precluding him from serving in *any* unit,'" was rejected in an unsigned order.[77]

There have been other, similar legal challenges made by DoD service members, all arguing that their religious objections to the vaccine should exempt them from the DoD mandate.[78] The plaintiffs in these lawsuits are generally represented by conservative nonprofit legal

---

[72] Sam Sachs, "Battle Lines Drawn in Vaccine Fight as Military Class-Action Lawsuit Contests Federal Mandate in Florida Court," *WFLA*, October 19, 2021.

[73] Liberty Counsel, "Navy SEAL 1 v. Austin Case Timeline," June 8, 2022; Sachs, 2021.

[74] Liberty Counsel, "Military, Federal Employees and Civilian Contractors Sue Biden," press release, October 15, 2021.

[75] Liberty Counsel, 2022.

[76] Heather Mongilio, "Supreme Court Rules Navy Can Reassign Unvaxxed SEALs," *USNI News*, March 28, 2022.

[77] Amy Howe, "With Three Conservatives Dissenting, Court Declines to Intervene on Behalf of Air Force Officer Who Won't Get Vaccinated," *SCOTUSblog*, April 18, 2022.

[78] For example, a lawsuit by 36 active duty airmen (Gina Dvorak and Ashly Richardson, "U.S. Airmen File Lawsuit Fighting Biden COVID-19 Vaccine Mandate," *WOWT*, March 8, 2022).

organizations, including the Alliance for Free Citizens, First Liberty Institute, and Liberty Counsel.[79]

To date, the courts have been uniformly friendly to the DoD COVID-19 vaccine mandate. With the Pfizer and Moderna vaccines no longer under EUA status, there is even less reason to think that the COVID-19 vaccine mandate will be overturned or that permanent administrative vaccine exemptions will be granted. Rather, in the future, the COVID-19 vaccination program will be more likely to be treated similarly to the general DoD vaccine program.

State-Level Policy Impact

Regarding vaccine mandates for service members (in particular, from the Army and Air National Guard), several states have challenged the military's vaccine mandate: Alaska, Idaho, Iowa, Mississippi, Nebraska, Oklahoma, Texas, and Wyoming. Alaska, Oklahoma, and Texas also filed lawsuits. The governors specifically were seeking to get Secretary of Defense Austin "not to enforce the mandate on National Guard troops."[80] In responding to the governors of these states, Austin highlighted the need "to maintain military readiness and the health of the force," and emphasized "that failure to get the vaccine 'may lead to a prohibition on the member's participation in drills and training' and could 'jeopardize the member's status in the National Guard.'"[81] In pressing the case for vaccination, Austin highlighted that "vaccination against COVID-19 is an essential military readiness requirement for all components and units of the military."[82]

To highlight the serious readiness implications of this noncompliance with the COVID-19 mandatory DoD vaccination policy, of the 20,000 Texas National Guard members, approximately 40 percent of the Army National Guard had refused the COVID-19 vaccination, citing "religious accommodation needs or otherwise," as of January 2022.[83] There would be serious readiness implications if 40 percent of the Texas National Guard were to be removed from the force through administrative or UCMJ actions or if that same 40 percent were to remain unvaccinated.

Countries Where U.S. Troops Are Stationed (e.g., Japan, Korea, Germany, Italy)

As we have seen previously, decisions about vaccination policy in specific theaters are based on guidance from the DoD Office of the Assistant Secretary of Defense for Health Affairs and the direction of the combatant commanders in their respective areas of responsibility. These

---

[79] Alliance for Free Citizens, homepage, undated; First Liberty Institute, homepage, undated; Liberty Counsel, homepage, undated.

[80] Baldor, 2022.

[81] Baldor, 2022.

[82] Baldor, 2022.

[83] Baldor, 2022.

decisions are normally made in accordance with competent U.S. health authorities and military commanders in coordination with host-nation health authorities.

One area where challenges could be seen regarding vaccines and testing is overseas travel, where testing, rather than vaccination status, was often used as a requirement for allowing entry into a country. This often resulted in previously vaccinated people with asymptomatic COVID-19 being quarantined based on the laws, policies, and protocols of the host nation or while transiting a country en route to or from the host nation.

Chapter 4. Case Studies: Other DoD Vaccine Campaigns and Mandates

In this chapter, we will consider vaccine programs within DoD that were implemented to respond to specific threats, deployments, or special work conditions that required more-specific vaccinations. Although the general vaccination program is well supported by military members, evidence suggests that specific vaccinations against potential biological warfare agents have a lower degree of acceptance.

Regarding the military's general vaccination program, Kwai-Cheung Chan, the U.S. General Accounting Office (GAO) Director for Applied Research and Methods, testified that, in a survey of National Guard and Reserve pilots and aircrew members, 74 percent believed that vaccinations were effective, and 60 percent saw immunizations as being safe.[84]

However, general views about the biological warfare immunizations did not follow this same trend, with 87 percent reporting "they would or probably would have concerns about safety if additional vaccines for other biological warfare agents were added to military immunization requirements."[85] In regard to the anthrax immunization program, 65 percent expressed "little or no support" for the program.[86]

Anthrax Vaccination

The development of an anthrax vaccine can be traced to the 1880s, when Louis Pasteur in France and W. S. Greenfield in the United Kingdom developed a heat-attenuated vaccine.[87] The Sterne strain discovered in the 1930s is considered "relatively avirulent" yet is sufficient "to stimulate a protective immune response."[88] It was used to develop a live attenuated spore vaccine, which was used to immunize livestock and humans, particularly those individuals likely to be exposed to anthrax through agriculture. This last point was important because the initial licensure of the vaccine was for protection against cutaneous anthrax rather than inhalational anthrax, which was deemed to be the threat to the force.

---

[84] Kwai-Cheung Chan, "Anthrax Vaccine: Preliminary Results of GAO's Survey of Guard/Reserve Pilots and Aircrew Members," testimony presented before the House Committee on Government Reform, U.S. General Accounting Office, GAO-01-92T, October 11, 2000, p. 2.

[85] Chan, 2000, p. 5.

[86] Chan, 2000, p. 2.

[87] W. D. Tigertt, "Anthrax. William Smith Greenfield, M.D., F.R.C.P., Professor Superintendent, the Brown Animal Sanatory Institution (1878–81): Concerning the Priority Due to Him for the Production of the First Vaccine Against Anthrax," *Journal of Hygiene*, Vol. 85, No. 3, December 1980.

[88] CDC, "Anthrax Sterne Strain (34F2) of Bacillus Anthracis," webpage, undated-b.

The anthrax vaccine adsorbed (AVA) used in the Anthrax Vaccine Immunization Program (AVIP) consisted of a six-dose regime administered over "18 months, with annual boosters thereafter."[89] It originally was licensed by the National Institutes of Health in 1970 (before the FDA became the licensing agency).

The DoD anthrax vaccination program began in December 1997 with the announcement by the Secretary of Defense that "all U.S. forces would be inoculated against the potential use of anthrax on the battlefield."[90] At the time of the announcement, the Secretary of Defense highlighted four preconditions for beginning the program, stipulating that

> immunizations would not begin until DoD (1) established a means of testing the vaccine over and above tests required by the Food and Drug Administration (FDA), (2) developed a system for tracking vaccinations, (3) approved operational and communication plans for the vaccination program, and (4) had an outside expert review the health and medical aspects of the program.[91]

When the preconditions were met, the mandatory AVIP began in August 1998 and included plans for vaccination of all 2.4 million active and reserve component service members. Units that were either deployed or scheduled to deploy to high-threat areas received priority for vaccination.

The lack of support for the anthrax vaccination program became evident almost immediately, specifically because of concerns about the safety and efficacy of the vaccine. One GAO report to Congress characterized the response as becoming an "increasing controversy," highlighting concerns about the prudence of relying on a single vaccine manufacturer and "the lack of studies on long-term safety and on human efficacy testing against inhaled anthrax."[92]

In contrast to the general military vaccination program, which is widely accepted as a precondition of service, the AVIP was not supported by 65 percent of the force. The GAO survey of National Guard and Reserve pilots and aircrews highlighted several concerns regarding the completeness, accuracy, timeliness, and potential bias of the information provided. Seventy-six percent of those surveyed indicated "they would not or probably would not take the shots if the anthrax immunization program were voluntary."[93]

Some service members expressed concerns, whether accurate or not, about adverse outcomes for those who began the anthrax vaccination course. In the survey, 42 percent stated they had received "one or more anthrax shots," with 86 percent "experiencing side effects or adverse

---

[89] Robert Roos, "Judge Orders DoD to Stop Requiring Anthrax Shots," Center for Infectious Disease Research and Policy, December 23, 2003.

[90] Chan, 2000, p. 3.

[91] GAO, *Medical Readiness: DOD Faces Challenges in Implementing Its Anthrax Vaccine Immunization Program*, GAO/NSIAD-00-36, October 1999, p. 3.

[92] GAO, 1999, p. 3.

[93] Chan, 2000, p. 2.

reactions."[94] A majority of those surveyed did not report symptoms, with some "citing fear of the loss of flight status" as a reason.[95]

By 2003, almost 1 million service members had been vaccinated using the AVA, yet service member concerns persisted. In a 2003 lawsuit seeking to halt the AVIP using the AVA, the judge said the vaccine had "never been specifically approved or labeled for use against inhalational anthrax, the main aim of the military vaccination program, as opposed to skin anthrax." The judge's ruling stated that "service members should not be vaccinated without their informed consent or a presidential waiver of the informed-consent requirement." The judge also indicated he was "persuaded that AVA is an investigational drug and a drug being used for an unapproved purpose."[96]

In defending the AVIP during the lawsuit, DoD officials identified only "105 serious adverse events among 830,000 anthrax vaccinees," yet the vaccine label indicates "an overall adverse-event rate of 5% to 35% and that six deaths have been blamed on the vaccine."[97] As a result of the lawsuit, an injunction was placed against the mandatory AVIP.

DoD responded by seeking EUA for those personnel "at high-risk for exposure to inhalation anthrax and asked the Food and Drug Administration (FDA) to approve."[98] EUA was granted by the FDA in January 2005, and the court then "modified its injunction to allow program resumption under EUA."[99] In October 2006, the Deputy Secretary of Defense approved a resumption of the AVIP.

The rollout of the AVIP resulted in safety and efficacy concerns and, eventually, a loss of confidence in the vaccine and the AVIP. These concerns cut across several stakeholders, from service members and families to commanders and Congress. One account describes the lasting effects of the AVIP as follows: "Service members' hesitancy to receive the anthrax vaccine left scars that are now affecting the COVID-19 vaccine mandate."[100]

Acceptability of the vaccine was negatively affected by its status. The original approval of the vaccine was not for aerosol exposure to anthrax, which is the likely method of dissemination for a state actor or bioterrorist and thus what would be most pertinent to military missions. The lawsuit and the subsequent designation of the vaccine as IND and later EUA led to a loss of confidence in the safety and efficacy of the AVA.

---

[94] Chan, 2000, p. 5.

[95] Chan, 2000, p. 3.

[96] Roos, 2003.

[97] Roos, 2003.

[98] War Related Illness and Injury Study Center, "Anthrax Vaccine: A Resource for Veterans, Service Members, and Their Families," U.S. Department of Veterans Affairs, updated August 2022.

[99] War Related Illness and Injury Study Center, 2022.

[100] Heather Mongilio, "U.S. Military Has Historically Struggled with Vaccine Hesitancy," *USNI News*, November 9, 2021.

Smallpox Vaccination

On December 13, 2002, the Under Secretary for Personnel and Readiness within the Office of the Secretary of Defense distributed an implementation memorandum for the Smallpox Vaccination Program (SVP). The memorandum established a three-stage implementation program that contained the following prioritization for vaccination: (1) smallpox response teams and hospital/clinic teams, (2) designated forces that constitute certain mission-critical capabilities, and (3) other U.S. forces, depending on circumstances.[101]

In describing the rationale for the SVP, the Air Force chief of staff described the vaccination program as "our Commanders' Force Protection Program against a deadly biological warfare agent,"[102] while the Army implementation memorandum to the force highlighted the need to "protect the health and safety of our personnel and preserve certain mission critical capabilities."[103] The Air Force chief in this memorandum further cautioned that "[s]uccessful implementation requires commanders to plan in advance for the operational, education, administration, logistics, and medical issues."[104]

In a report to Congress titled *Review of the Implementation of the Military Program*, GAO evaluated the execution of the DoD portion of the national SVP. The report highlighted the benefits of the DoD approach of implementing the program in stages, allowing the department to carefully monitor potential adverse reactions and adjust as necessary to ensure understanding of the program. The use of the first stage, which served as a pilot program for the larger DoD SVP, provided an opportunity to learn during the initial implementation of the program.[105]

The Army served as the executive agent for DoD. This organizational delineation provided a responsible element to oversee the progress toward the national and DoD goals. It also contributed to minimizing the amount of vaccine that was wasted or contaminated or that experienced a loss of potency.[106]

Unlike with the anthrax vaccination program, the SVP was initially targeted to vaccinate those in stage one (smallpox response teams and hospital/clinic teams) and those elements of stage two that were in CENTCOM's area of responsibility (designated forces that constitute

---

[101] David S. C. Chu, Under Secretary of Defense for Personnel and Readiness, "Policy on Administrative Issues Related to Smallpox Vaccination Program (SVP)," memorandum, December 13, 2002.

[102] John P. Jumper, Air Force Chief of Staff, "Air Force Implementation of the Smallpox Vaccination Program," memorandum, January 7, 2003.

[103] John M. Keane, Army Vice Chief of Staff, "Army Smallpox Vaccination Implementation Plan," memorandum, January 10, 2003.

[104] Jumper, 2003.

[105] GAO, *Smallpox Vaccination: Implementation of National Program Faces Challenges*, GAO-03-578, April 2003a.

[106] GAO, 2003a.

certain mission-critical capabilities). The memorandum explicitly allowed for expanding the program priorities "at a later date."[107]

Furthermore, the memorandum established the cohort of affected personnel, including military personnel, DoD civilian personnel identified as emergency-essential, contractor personnel performing mission-essential services, other personnel characterized as alert forces, and other civilian employees who are designated members of a smallpox response team.[108]

The services were directed to develop plans to administer the smallpox vaccinations to approved personnel. The planning required developing operational plans for implementing the SVP, as well as education and training for all personnel subject to the program and tracking systems. Exemptions were possible, as was request for including other personnel in the SVP. Exemptions could be administrative or medical and could, but did not necessarily, change a person's deployability status. As highlighted in the GAO memorandum, DoD also established guidelines for people not eligible to receive the vaccine, which included (1) personnel with allergies to the smallpox vaccine, those who were breastfeeding, and those who had certain cardiac conditions; (2) personnel with a compromised immune system, eczema or atopic dermatitis, active skin disease (such as psoriasis), or those who were pregnant; or (3) personnel living with someone who had one or more of these four contraindications.

The GAO report can best be summarized by the finding that "DOD Facilitated Its Smallpox Vaccination Program by Ensuring the Availability of the Vaccine and by Educating Its Personnel."[109] We would add that the targeting of mission-oriented groups also created a positive understanding of why those designated to receive the vaccines were selected. Other factors that contributed to the acceptability of the SVP include a vaccine that was FDA approved and the care taken to identify at-risk populations (and potential dangers to their families) to ensure that they did not take the vaccine.

By October 2003, more than 500,000 personnel across the five services (including the Coast Guard) had been vaccinated. Only 184 people who had received the smallpox vaccine had "noteworthy adverse reactions."[110] This is made even more remarkable given that the version of the vaccine during this period "contains a live virus that can be spread from a vaccinee" to others.[111] It implies that the screening that was done of those receiving the vaccination exempted those who might have adverse reactions to the smallpox vaccine.

---

[107] Chu, 2002.

[108] Chu, 2002.

[109] GAO, "Small Pox Vaccination: Review of the Implementation of the Military Program," memorandum to Senate Committee on Governmental Affairs Chairman Susan M. Collins, GAO-04-215R, December 1, 2003b, p. 8.

[110] GAO, 2003b, p. 7.

[111] GAO, 2003b, p. 6.

The ACAM2000 smallpox vaccine is now available, which does not use live virus and is therefore much safer to use.[112] Special groups and soldiers deployed to designated theaters routinely get the smallpox vaccine.

The Gulf War

Although military personnel typically get vaccinations against endemic diseases prior to deployments, concerns about Saddam Hussein's weapons of mass destruction (WMD) programs resulted in several medical countermeasures and prophylaxis being deployed to the theater in the event of a nuclear, chemical, or biological attack or exposure to these substances on the battlefield.

The "standard series of inoculations against infectious diseases provided to any U.S. citizen traveling to the Gulf (including yellow fever, typhoid, cholera, hepatitis B, meningitis, whooping cough, polio, tetanus)" was also provided to deployed service members.[113]

Some pre- and post-exposure prophylaxis and vaccines were offered to soldiers but were not uniformly available to deployed forces. Soldiers carried atropine injections in the event of exposure to chemical nerve agents. Pyridostigmine bromide was offered as pre-exposure prophylaxis for nerve agent exposure as well. An anthrax vaccine was also offered optionally for deployed soldiers.[114]

One account from the Institute of Medicine stated,

> It is estimated that 310,680 doses of the anthrax vaccine licensed by the Food and Drug Administration (FDA) were distributed to the Gulf War theatre and that 150,000 U.S. troops received at least one anthrax vaccination. . . . Approximately 137,850 doses of botulinum toxoid were sent to the Gulf, and it is estimated that 8,000 individuals were vaccinated.[115]

Although there is no evidence to establish a causal link between a cluster of long-term health problems experienced by service members and the vaccinations they received leading up to their Gulf War service, concerns about environmental exposures continue to plague a small population of those service members who were deployed to the Gulf War in 1990–1991. The U.S. Department of Veterans Affairs offers the following disclaimer in one of its publications: "There is inadequate or insufficient evidence to determine whether an association does or does not exist between multiple vaccinations and long-term adverse health problems."[116] The Veterans Benefits Administration describes these "unexplained illnesses" as "a cluster of medically unexplained

---

[112] CDC, "Smallpox: Vaccines," webpage, undated-g.

[113] U.S. Department of Veterans Affairs, "Vaccinations and Gulf War Veterans," webpage, undated-b.

[114] U.S. Department of Veterans Affairs, undated-b.

[115] Carolyn E. Fulco, Catharyn T. Liverman, and Harold C. Sox, eds., *Gulf War and Health*: Vol. 1, *Depleted Uranium, Sarin, Pyridostigmine Bromide, Vaccines*, National Academy Press, 2000, pp. 267–268.

[116] U.S. Department of Veterans Affairs, undated-b.

chronic symptoms that can include fatigue, headaches, joint pain, indigestion, insomnia, dizziness, respiratory disorders, and memory problems."[117]

Although Iraq had WMD programs and had chemical weapons stockpiled, there is no evidence of the use of these munitions against coalition forces. There were, however, inadvertent chemical exposures to coalition forces during the destruction of these munitions at the end of hostilities.[118]

"Mandates" as Provision of Work

Certain military, civilian, or contractor positions that support DoD are required to have vaccinations that exceed the normal requirements. These positions include individuals who might have a higher risk of being exposed to biological agents because of the provisions of their work. Included personnel are those who work in high-containment biological laboratories, certain law enforcement officials, and medical personnel, to name a few special categories. We highlight these personnel as a special category, but, as the delineation of personnel groups in the smallpox section above indicates, the number of people in these programs can expand and contract based on mission requirements. The requirement for special vaccinations is therefore directly linked to the work that one will be performing.

For example, researchers who are working with select agents should be vaccinated against any pathogens they are likely to encounter during the course of their research. The type of pathogen will also delineate the level of precautions that researchers will need to take. Pathogens for which there are no approved treatments or vaccines should be worked with only in a high-containment Biological Safety Level 4 facility.[119] As an example, if a researcher will be working with a pathogen such as Ebola in a high-containment facility, the Ebola vaccine would be required, which was approved by the FDA in December 2019.[120] This guidance would pertain to all personnel, whether military, DoD civilian, or contractor.

Special operations forces, certain members of the 20th Support Command (Chemical Biological, Radiological, Nuclear, Explosive) with unique missions in countering WMD, and WMD Civil Support Teams (which are military units that support state governors) would also likely have requirements for vaccination that exceed the nine immunizations that are required for

---

[117] U.S. Department of Veterans Affairs, "Gulf War Veterans' Medically Unexplained Illnesses," webpage, undated-a.

[118] Daniel M. Gerstein, the lead author of this report, served with the 3rd Armored Division in Operations Desert Shield and Desert Storm. At the end of hostilities, soldiers clearing the munitions bunkers were exposed to what was determined to be mustard agent.

[119] CDC, "High Containment Laboratories at CDC—Fifty Years of Excellence," webpage, undated-e.

[120] CDC, "Ebola Vaccine: Information About ERVEBO," webpage, undated-d.

all military personnel, active duty and reserve, as part of the adult routine schedule or upon accession.[121]

Depending on the mission and likely threats to be encountered, people who need vaccines as a provision of work may be required to agree to be vaccinated with IND or EUA vaccines in addition to approved vaccines. Those who do not voluntarily accept one of these vaccines needed for a particular mission would likely be removed from that mission.

---

[121] Headquarters, Departments of the Army, the Navy, the Air Force, and the Coast Guard, 2013, p. 11.

Chapter 5. Observations and Conclusions

In this chapter, we present an exploratory framework based on our limited observations and analysis.

We propose indicators based on our analysis that allowed us to both differentiate between the acceptability of the various vaccine programs and identify concerns that surfaced in the development of vaccine mandates for each. We believe that the following six key attributes should be considered in any future DoD vaccination campaign: (1) approval status of vaccine, (2) targeting groups for vaccines, (3) consistent messaging, (4) instilling confidence in the technology, (5) disinformation surrounding the vaccine, and (6) perceived care in making decisions about mandates.

Observations and Assessments

In seeking to draw conclusions, we compared the vaccination campaigns for anthrax, smallpox, and COVID-19. We did not seek to compare the Gulf War or mandates as a provision of work with the three campaigns because there are significant differences in these cases that make direct comparisons challenging. Our framework, which includes the six criteria and associated rating scales for each, is provided in Table 5.1. To illustrate the potential of this framework, we assessed the three vaccination campaigns using the information gleaned in the case studies. The results are plotted in Figure 5.1.

Approval status relates to where the vaccine is in its life cycle, which could range from full approval to uncertainty surrounding its approval. The case of the anthrax vaccine is instructive for understanding what this uncertainty might entail. The anthrax vaccine, while approved for treatment of cutaneous anthrax cases, was never approved for inhalational anthrax, which was the primary concern for establishing the AVIP.

The *targeting of certain groups* for vaccination or to receive priority is the second indicator. More-targeted campaigns that related vaccination requirements to a service member's specific duties were deemed more acceptable. For example, the SVP employed a pilot program, with the highest-priority personnel as the first recipients.

The third indicator pertains to the *messaging employed* in discussing the vaccine with its intended audience. Clear, unambiguous messaging translated to higher acceptability, whereas mixed messages were associated with a lower degree of acceptability.

Technology status, the fourth indicator, is used to identify where the technology was in its life cycle. If a vaccine was fully approved and used previously (for its intended purpose), it was seen as more acceptable, whereas vaccines that were EUA or IND were more susceptible to service members raising concerns.

The fifth attribute is *disinformation surrounding the vaccine.* This could include questions related to the safety and efficacy of the vaccine. The disinformation could be based on a lack of a track record, as in the case of the COVID-19 messenger RNA technology, or issues surfacing about previous uses of the vaccine, as in the case of the AVIP, which had been erroneously linked with Gulf War Syndrome.

The sixth and final attribute is DoD's *perceived care* in making decisions about the vaccinations, including the possibility of exemptions based on administrative, medical, or other (e.g., religious) considerations. Service members' perceptions of care in regard to DoD's decisions about the campaign could come from a variety of approaches, from running pilot programs (as in the case of the SVP) to the accurate messaging and tamping down on disinformation immediately.

Table 5.1. Proposed Rating Scale for Attributes

Indicator Level	Approval Status	Targeted Groups	Consistent Messaging	Technology	Disinformation	Perceived Care
5	Full	High	Fully	In use	None	High
4	EUA	Moderate	Moderate	Proven	Some	Significant
3	IND	Some	Some	Early use only	Moderate	Some
2	Clinical trials	Limited	Limited	New	High	Limited
1	Uncertain	None	None	Emerging	Overwhelming	None

The six evaluation categories logically fit into three larger bins: (1) the state of the vaccine's technological development, which includes approval status and technology status, (2) the degree of rigor in DoD's messaging about the vaccine's utility, which includes consistent messaging and countering disinformation, and (3) the extent of DoD's strategic deployment of the vaccine campaign, which includes targeted groups and perceived care.

Figure 5.1. Comparison of Anthrax, Smallpox, and COVID-19 Vaccine Campaigns

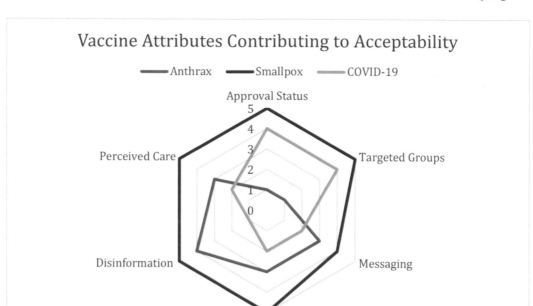

In our comparison of the anthrax, smallpox, and COVID-19 vaccine campaigns, the SVP was assessed to be the most effective, with the least amount of controversy. The vaccine was fully approved for use and had been in use for decades. DoD leadership developed a highly targeted vaccination strategy that demonstrated the need for and urgency of vaccinating specific populations. The use of a pilot program allowed for learning lessons, detailed messaging, and demonstrating prudence in the campaign. The establishment of rational exemptions based on objective (and documented) criteria also increased the acceptability of the vaccine.

The anthrax vaccination program, in contrast, came under fire by stakeholders almost immediately. The AVIP campaign was not targeted and used a vaccine that was intended for cutaneous anthrax exposures: It was not intended to address the inhalational anthrax threat that the campaign was meant to address. Furthermore, the AVIP had to be halted in response to legal challenges; once these were addressed, the AVIP was resumed. The messaging of the AVIP campaign was also not effective. Offering a voluntary anthrax vaccine during the Gulf War for deployed service members likely confused the broader uniformed population, who were intended to receive the vaccine as part of the AVIP. Additionally, concerns about illnesses of unknown origin affecting Gulf War veterans contributed to vaccine hesitancy.

In comparing the COVID-19 vaccine program with the AVIP and SVP, we remind the reader that the COVID-19 vaccine was intended for the majority of the population of the United States, whereas the AVIP and SVP vaccines were intended for DoD and other specialized populations who had the potential to become exposed to anthrax or smallpox during the course of their work, whether in health care, emergency management, or law enforcement or in uniform.

The COVID-19 vaccine has the distinction of being the most rapid program ever to result in a vaccine. In less than a year, the vaccine was developed, was put through clinical trials, and received EUA approval by the FDA, which allowed it to be administered to civilian and military populations. The urgency surrounding the COVID-19 vaccine program led policymakers and researchers to closely monitor the development of the vaccine candidates and to promote (we might even say overpromote) the vaccines while raising expectations for safety and efficacy.

During the COVID-19 pandemic, the response to the disease became highly politicized, and the vaccine was no exception. Some distributed false information about the use of fetal tissue in developing the vaccine. Others promoted conspiracy theories about microchips implanted through the administering of the vaccine. The emphasis on the speed of development caused some to express concerns about the safety of the vaccine. A very small group among those who had taken either one of the two messenger RNA vaccines or the J&J adenovirus vaccine reported adverse reactions. The J&J vaccine concerns were well documented and included a variety of symptoms, such as myocarditis and irregular blood clotting, which led to the FDA revising the guidance on individuals who should abstain from taking this vaccine in favor of one of the two messenger RNA immunizations.

Recommendations

Overall, the military's COVID-19 vaccination program has been successful, with vaccination of the force in the high 90 percent range for most populations, which is higher than for the general U.S. population as of this writing. The notable exceptions are the U.S. Army National Guard and Reserves: Even as of June 2022, these groups had lower rates of COVID-19 vaccination than the rest of the uniformed military, with 12 percent and 10 percent remaining unvaccinated. All of these rates—including the National Guard and Reserves—exceeded national vaccination rates.[122] Still, more than 8,400 service members have refused the COVID-19 vaccine and were discharged as a result.[123]

DoD's COVID-19 vaccination program was linked to and followed the national COVID-19 vaccine development, approval, and timelines. As a result, DoD and its service members expressed many of the same concerns as the civilian population.

In terms of tracking mechanisms, there are opportunities for improvement. We identified a lack of consistency across the services for tracking and recording information on vaccine administration as a concern, along with the lack of consistency in terms of granting exemptions. The 2022 National Defense Authorization Act recognizes these shortcomings and directs the department to develop a uniform approach to vaccination tracking and recording.

---

[122] CDC, "COVID Data Tracker: COVID-19 Vaccinations in the United States," updated March 9, 2023.

[123] Paul D. Shinkman, "Pentagon: No Back Pay to Troops Discharged for Refusing COVID-19 Vaccine," *U.S. News & World Report*, January 17, 2023.

We believe that our exploratory framework for considering vaccine acceptability—including the attributes that are identified in Table 5.1—could provide an important basis for thinking about how to manage future DoD vaccination campaigns. Although not all of the attributes are within the purview of the department, thinking about ways to mitigate those that are under DoD control and taking actions to lessen the impact of the other attributes could provide benefits for the long-term acceptability of any future vaccination program.

Highly targeted vaccination campaigns with consistent messaging that relates vaccination requirements to force health protection and mission readiness are essential.

We also have the following specific recommendations that could improve DoD's capacity for managing and tracking future vaccination campaigns:

- *Develop a department-wide tracking mechanism for vaccinations.* Although a decentralized approach to implementing the vaccine programs across the military services provides flexibility in how the services manage their workforce, operational readiness, and force health protection, having a consolidated, department-wide view of the status of vaccinations would be useful.
- *Employ a structured framework for development and implementation of future vaccination campaign plans.* As discussed, we believe that our exploratory framework could provide the basis for such a structured approach.
- *For future vaccination campaigns, seek to prioritize timely, accurate strategic communications based on factual information.* Although this messaging did occur for the COVID-19 vaccine, additional emphasis could lead to improved understanding of the vaccine and, ultimately, its acceptance across the force. Such communications could also be targeted to particular populations, such as the U.S. Army National Guard and Reserves, that have demonstrated less willingness to get the vaccines.

Abbreviations

ACIP	Advisory Committee on Immunization Practices
AVA	anthrax vaccine adsorbed
AVIP	Anthrax Vaccine Immunization Program
AWOL	absent without leave
CDC	Centers for Disease Control and Prevention
CENTCOM	U.S. Central Command
COVID-19	coronavirus disease 2019
DoD	Department of Defense
EUA	Emergency Use Authorization
FDA	Food and Drug Administration
GAO	U.S. General Accounting Office
HHS	Department of Health and Human Services
IND	Investigational New Drug
J&J	Johnson & Johnson
SRP	soldier readiness processing
SVP	Smallpox Vaccination Program
UCMJ	Uniform Code of Military Justice
WMD	weapons of mass destruction

References

Aker, Janet A., "More Than 95% of Active Duty Have Received COVID-19 Vaccine," Defense Health Agency, October 15, 2021.

Alliance for Free Citizens, homepage, undated. As of March 10, 2023:
https://www.allianceforfreecitizens.org

Baldor, Lolita C., "Austin to Governors: Guard Troops Must Get COVID-19 Vaccine," Associated Press, January 31, 2022.

Billingsley, Alyssa, "FDA COVID-19 Vaccine Approval: Live Updates on Pfizer, Moderna, and J&J Vaccines," GoodRx Health, updated May 20, 2022.

Brothers, Will, "A Timeline of COVID-19 Vaccine Development," BioSpace, December 3, 2020.

Byerly, Carol R., "War Losses (USA)," in Ute Daniel, Peter Gatrell, Oliver Janz, Heather Jones, Jennifer Keene, Alan Kramer, and Bill Nasson, eds., *1914–1918 Online: International Encyclopedia of the First World War*, Freie Universität Berlin, 2014.

CDC—*See* Centers for Disease Control and Prevention.

CENTCOM—*See* U.S. Central Command.

Centers for Disease Control and Prevention, "Advisory Committee on Immunization Practices (ACIP): General Committee-Related Information," webpage, undated-a. As of March 10, 2023:
https://www.cdc.gov/vaccines/acip/committee/index.html

Centers for Disease Control and Prevention, "Anthrax Sterne Strain (34F2) of Bacillus Anthracis," webpage, undated-b. As of May 6, 2022:
https://www.cdc.gov/anthrax/resources/anthrax-sterne-strain.html

Centers for Disease Control and Prevention, "COVID-19 Vaccine Emergency Use Authorization (EUA) Fact Sheets for Recipients and Caregivers," webpage, undated-c. As of May 5, 2022:
https://www.cdc.gov/vaccines/covid-19/eua/index.html

Centers for Disease Control and Prevention, "Ebola Vaccine: Information About ERVEBO," webpage, undated-d. As of March 10, 2023:
https://www.cdc.gov/vhf/ebola/clinicians/vaccine/index.html

Centers for Disease Control and Prevention, "High Containment Laboratories at CDC—Fifty Years of Excellence," webpage, undated-e. As of March 10, 2023:
https://www.cdc.gov/ncezid/dhcpp/hcl-50/high-containment-laboratories.html

Centers for Disease Control and Prevention, "Janssen (Johnson & Johnson) COVID-19 Vaccine," webpage, undated-f. As of March 10, 2023:
https://www.cdc.gov/vaccines/covid-19/info-by-product/janssen/index.html

Centers for Disease Control and Prevention, "Smallpox: Vaccines," webpage, undated-g. As of May 6, 2022:
https://www.cdc.gov/smallpox/clinicians/vaccines.html

Centers for Disease Control and Prevention, "COVID Data Tracker: COVID-19 Vaccinations in the United States," updated March 9, 2023. As of March 10, 2023:
https://covid.cdc.gov/covid-data-tracker/#vaccinations_vacc-people-additional-dose-totalpop

Chan, Kwai-Cheung, "Anthrax Vaccine: Preliminary Results of GAO's Survey of Guard/Reserve Pilots and Aircrew Members," testimony presented before the House Committee on Government Reform, U.S. General Accounting Office, GAO-01-92T, October 11, 2000.

Christensen, Paul A., Randall J. Olsen, S. Wesley Long, Sishir Subedi, James J. Davis, Parsa Hodjat, Debbie R. Walley, Jacob C. Kinskey, Matthew Ojeda Saavedra, Layne Pruitt, et al., "Delta Variants of SARS-CoV-2 Cause Significantly Increased Vaccine Breakthrough COVID-19 Cases in Houston, Texas," *American Journal of Pathology*, Vol. 192, No. 2, February 2022.

Chu, David S. C., Under Secretary of Defense for Personnel and Readiness, "Policy on Administrative Issues Related to Smallpox Vaccination Program (SVP)," memorandum, December 13, 2002.

Cirillo, Vincent J., "Two Faces of Death: Fatalities from Disease and Combat in America's Principal Wars, 1775 to Present," *Perspectives in Biology and Medicine*, Vol. 51, No. 1, Winter 2008.

Cisneros, Gilbert R., Jr., Under Secretary of Defense for Personnel and Readiness, "Force Health Protection Guidance (Supplement 23) Revision 1—Department of Defense Guidance for Coronavirus Disease 2019 Vaccination Attestation, Screening Testing, and Vaccination Verification," memorandum for senior Pentagon leadership, commanders of the combatant commands, and defense agency and DoD field activity directors, October 18, 2021.

College of Physicians of Philadelphia, "U.S. Military and Vaccine History," webpage, undated. As of May 5, 2022:
https://historyofvaccines.org/vaccines-101/how-are-vaccines-made/us-military-and-vaccine-history

Defense Health Agency, "Vaccine Recommendations by AOR," webpage, undated. As of March 10, 2023:
https://www.health.mil/Military-Health-Topics/Health-Readiness/Immunization-Healthcare/Vaccine-Recommendations/Vaccine-Recommendations-by-AOR

Delgado, Carla, "More Hospitals Are Now Mandating COVID-19 Vaccines for Healthcare Workers," Verywell Health, July 30, 2021.

Department of Defense, "Coronavirus: DOD Response," webpage, undated. As of March 10, 2023:
https://www.defense.gov/Spotlights/Coronavirus-DOD-Response/DOD-Response-Ti-/

Department of Defense, "Mandatory Coronavirus Disease 2019 Vaccination of DoD Civilian Employees," press release, October 4, 2021.

Department of Defense, "Consolidated Department of Defense Coronavirus Disease 2019 Force Health Protection Guidance," press release, April 6, 2022.

Department of Defense Instruction 6205.02, *DoD Immunization Program*, U.S. Department of Defense, July 23, 2019.

Deputy Secretary of Defense, "Clarifying Guidance for Smallpox and Anthrax Vaccine Immunization Program," memorandum, November 12, 2015.

DoD—*See* Department of Defense.

Doherty, Peter C., "Stealth Attack: Infection and Disease on the Battlefield," *The Conversation*, June 8, 2015.

Dvorak, Gina, and Ashly Richardson, "U.S. Airmen File Lawsuit Fighting Biden COVID-19 Vaccine Mandate," *WOWT*, March 8, 2022.

Edwards, Erika, "FDA Adds Warning to J&J Vaccine for Possible Link to Rare Neurological Disorder," *NBC News*, July 12, 2021.

First Liberty Institute, homepage, undated. As of March 10, 2023:
https://firstliberty.org

Food and Drug Administration, "Vaccines," webpage, undated. As of May 5, 2022:
https://www.fda.gov/vaccines-blood-biologics/vaccines

Fort Stewart-Hunter Army Airfield, "Soldier Readiness Processing," webpage, undated. As of March 10, 2023:
https://home.army.mil/stewart/index.php/about/Garrison/DHR/SRP

Fulco, Carolyn E., Catharyn T. Liverman, and Harold C. Sox, eds., *Gulf War and Health*: Vol. 1, *Depleted Uranium, Sarin, Pyridostigmine Bromide, Vaccines*, National Academy Press, 2000.

GAO—*See* U.S. General Accounting Office.

Hamel, Liz, Lunna Lopes, Grace Sparks, Ashley Kirzinger, Audrey Kearney, Mellisha Stokes, and Mollyann Brodie, "KFF COVID-19 Vaccine Monitor: September 2021," Kaiser Family Foundation, September 28, 2021.

Headquarters, Departments of the Army, the Navy, the Air Force, and the Coast Guard, *Immunizations and Chemoprophylaxis for the Prevention of Infectious Diseases*, October 7, 2013.

Horton, Alex, "As Army Deadline Nears, About 60,000 Part-Time Soldiers Unvaccinated," *Washington Post*, June 24, 2022.

Howe, Amy, "With Three Conservatives Dissenting, Court Declines to Intervene on Behalf of Air Force Officer Who Won't Get Vaccinated," *SCOTUSblog*, April 18, 2022.

I Corps Regulation 600-8-101, *Soldier Readiness Program (SRP)*, Headquarters, I Corps, undated.

J&J—*See* Johnson & Johnson.

Johnson & Johnson, "Johnson & Johnson COVID-19 Vaccine Authorized by U.S. FDA for Emergency Use—First Single-Shot Vaccine in Fight Against Global Pandemic," press release, February 27, 2021

Jumper, John P., Air Force Chief of Staff, "Air Force Implementation of the Smallpox Vaccination Program," memorandum, January 7, 2003.

Keane, John M., Army Vice Chief of Staff, "Army Smallpox Vaccination Implementation Plan," memorandum, January 10, 2003.

Liberty Counsel, homepage, undated. As of March 10, 2023:
https://lc.org

Liberty Counsel, "Military, Federal Employees and Civilian Contractors Sue Biden," press release, October 15, 2021.

Liberty Counsel, "Navy SEAL 1 v. Austin Case Timeline," June 8, 2022.

MacMillan, Carrie, "Emergency Use Authorization vs. Full FDA Approval: What's the Difference?" Yale Medicine, March 7, 2022.

Mandal, Ananya, "COVID-19 Outbreak on an American Aircraft Carrier: A Case Study in Transmission," News Medical, November 16, 2020.

Mendez, Bryce H. P., "Defense Health Primer: Military Vaccinations," Congressional Research Service, IF11816, updated August 6, 2021a.

Mendez, Bryce H. P., "The Military's COVID-19 Vaccination Mandate," Congressional Research Service, IN11764, updated November 8, 2021b.

Military Health System, homepage, undated. As of March 10, 2023: https://www.health.mil

Mongilio, Heather, "U.S. Military Has Historically Struggled with Vaccine Hesitancy," *USNI News*, November 9, 2021.

Mongilio, Heather, "Supreme Court Rules Navy Can Reassign Unvaxxed SEALs," *USNI News*, March 28, 2022.

National Academies of Sciences, Engineering, and Medicine, "National Academies Release Draft Framework for Equitable Allocation of a COVID-19 Vaccine, Seek Public Comment," press release, September 1, 2020a.

National Academies of Sciences, Engineering, and Medicine, "National Academies Release Framework for Equitable Allocation of a COVID-19 Vaccine for Adoption by HHS, State, Tribal, Local, and Territorial Authorities," press release, October 2, 2020b.

Nix, Elizabeth, "Tuskegee Experiment: The Infamous Syphilis Study," History, December 15, 2020.

Public Law 117-81, National Defense Authorization Act for Fiscal Year 2022, December 27, 2021.

Riley, Pete, Michal Ben-Nun, James Turtle, David Bacon, Akeisha N. Owens, and Steven Riley, "COVID-19: On the Disparity in Outcomes Between Military and Civilian Populations," *Military Medicine*, Vol. 188, No. 1–2, January–February 2023.

Roos, Robert, "Judge Orders DoD to Stop Requiring Anthrax Shots," Center for Infectious Disease Research and Policy, December 23, 2003.

Sachs, Sam, "Battle Lines Drawn in Vaccine Fight as Military Class-Action Lawsuit Contests Federal Mandate in Florida Court," *WFLA*, October 19, 2021.

Shinkman, Paul D., "Pentagon: No Back Pay to Troops Discharged for Refusing COVID-19 Vaccine," *U.S. News & World Report*, January 17, 2023.

Tigertt, W. D., "Anthrax. William Smith Greenfield, M.D., F.R.C.P., Professor Superintendent, the Brown Animal Sanatory Institution (1878–81): Concerning the Priority Due to Him for the Production of the First Vaccine Against Anthrax," *Journal of Hygiene*, Vol. 85, No. 3, December 1980.

USAFacts, "US Coronavirus Vaccine Tracker: What's the Nation's Progress on Vaccinations?" webpage, undated. As of May 2022: https://usafacts.org/visualizations/covid-vaccine-tracker-states/

U.S. Central Command, "USCENTCOM 091923Z Apr 20 Mod Fifteen to USCENTCOM Individual Protection and Individual-Unit Deployment Policy," 2020.

U.S. Department of Veterans Affairs, "Gulf War Veterans' Medically Unexplained Illnesses," webpage, undated-a. As of May 6, 2022:
https://www.publichealth.va.gov/exposures/gulfwar/medically-unexplained-illness.asp

U.S. Department of Veterans Affairs, "Vaccinations and Gulf War Veterans," webpage, undated-b. As of May 6, 2022:
https://www.publichealth.va.gov/exposures/gulfwar/sources/vaccinations.asp

U.S. General Accounting Office, *Medical Readiness: DOD Faces Challenges in Implementing Its Anthrax Vaccine Immunization Program*, GAO/NSIAD-00-36, October 1999.

U.S. General Accounting Office, *Smallpox Vaccination: Implementation of National Program Faces Challenges*, GAO-03-578, April 2003a.

U.S. General Accounting Office, "Small Pox Vaccination: Review of the Implementation of the Military Program," memorandum to Senate Committee on Governmental Affairs Chairman Susan M. Collins, GAO-04-215R, December 1, 2003b.

U.S. Government Accountability Office, *Operation Warp Speed: Accelerated COVID-19 Vaccine Development Status and Efforts to Address Manufacturing Challenges*, GAO-21-319, February 11, 2021.

Van Beusekom, Mary, "COVID-19 Spread Freely Aboard USS Theodore Roosevelt, Report Shows," Center for Infectious Disease Research and Policy, October 1, 2020.

War Related Illness and Injury Study Center, "Anthrax Vaccine: A Resource for Veterans, Service Members, and Their Families," U.S. Department of Veterans Affairs, updated August 2022.

White House, "Executive Order on Requiring Coronavirus Disease 2019 Vaccination for Federal Employees," September 9, 2021.